SAVE YOUR BREATH

THE "STRESS-FREE" GUIDE ON OVERCOMING NICOTINE ADDICTION

SONIA M SHEEHAN

ISBN – 13:9781927677735

DEDICATION

THIS BOOK IS DEDICATED TO MY HUSBAND, GLEN.

THANK YOU FOR ALL OF YOUR PATIENCE AND SUPPORT.

LOVE ALWAYS, SONIA.

ALSO TO MY NIECE, CAITLYN,

AND NEPHEWS, MYLES AND BAILEY,

WHO I HOPE NEVER START SMOKING.

LOVE ALWAYS, AUNTIE SONIA.

SONIA SHEEHAN

FOREWORD

I've helped publish many guides and authorities' books over the past decade, and have worked with many talented authors, but none yet has shown more dedication to helping others than Sonia Sheehan. Sonia is your expert personal trainer to stop smoking. She's done it herself, and she knows exactly how to guide you through your own journey toward becoming a non-smoker. Every time you might hit a block during your journey, Sonia is right there with you. Sonia was a smoker for twenty-seven years before she finally stopped; she's been there herself, and she knows exactly the right tool and the perfect tip to help you work through your obstacle and become closer to stopping smoking forever.

Many people have had struggles with smoking in

their past and overcome them, but most of them have never quite managed to share the lessons they learned in that process. If they had ever attempted to share what they learned, it would have never been as succinct as how Sonia puts it in this book. Sonia had to try quitting over and over again before she figured out what she was doing wrong and finally succeeded.

This book isn't about all the things she did wrong (although she does share some of her failures with her readers). It is about all the things she did *right* before she was able to finally put the butt out forever and proudly call herself a non-smoker. It's about how not to do it wrong. It's not about setting quit dates, or getting a nicotine patch. It's not about paying the high prices for different sorts of therapies. Sonia presents her own method for stopping smoking that worked for her, and will most likely be the exact method that will help you succeed in your quest as well.

When you walk into the self-help aisle of the bookstore or search the Internet, looking for "how to quit smoking," you will surely find an abundance of resources at your hands. But I can assure you, I've browsed through many of them, and none contain the expert knowledge and lived experiences that Sonia details in this book. These other books and blogs you'll find are often written based on scare tactics, or as bibles of statistics on smoking and health problems, or as a collection of tips and advices, or just simply as one person's story and struggles with stopping smoking. This book is none of that, but all of that at the same time. Sonia seamlessly weaves her own tales and battles throughout the book as she gives you her learned advice and her tried-and-true strategies for butting out, while providing just enough facts about smoking to keep you grounded about why you might want to stop.

If you are thinking of stopping smoking, for the very first time or the very final time, then you have got yourself the right book, written by the right person. Sonia will convince you that anyone can have the strength, power, and capacity to stop smoking forever.

Raymond Aaron

New York Times Best Selling Author

Contents

SONIA SHEEHAN

A Personal Note from the Author

Dear reader, my name is Sonia Sheehan, and I want to outline the reasons I am writing this book and how it will be presented.

I want to explain to you there are other methods and ways to stop smoking, other than the ones we have been told about previously by the so-called experts. You are an individual; therefore you need your own system to stop smoking, in your own time and on your own terms. We can't all do it the same way, and this book outlines how you can devise your own system and work at your own stress-free pace to eventually become totally nicotine-free.

This book is about how I finally became nicotine-free after smoking cigarettes for 27 years. It's about how I coped, what barriers I came up against during that period of my life and, especially, what I learned along the way. I know I don't have to try and scare you to stop smoking, we all know that smoking isn't good for us, that it shortens our lives, and it harms others around us. I want to be frank and suggest a method that you could adopt to become a happy non-smoker like me. I am so excited about this book, because I firmly believe it *will* help others stop. I hope you find it inspirational and find motivation within you to achieve your "wants." I appreciate that you have decided to read my book and I encourage you to give me any feedback, and to tell me your story. I look forward to hearing from you. Please visit my website: www.saveyourbreathbook.com.

Thank you very much, and I wish you all the success in your endeavors to achieve nicotine freedom.

Chapter 1

Getting Hooked, Line and Sinker.......

I started smoking cigarettes at the naïve age of 13, totally unaware of the significance and what the consequences would be for the next 27 years.

Those days, everyone smoked. My father, my best friend's parents, my neighbors – it was everywhere. By grade eight, my friends and I started to notice the older kids who smoked, and the girls who would get their cigarettes lit by their older boyfriends. And then people in our grade started to smoke too. This was the 1980's in Queensland, Australia.

One afternoon whilst at my friend's place, we decided that it was our turn to try smoking. We wanted to see if we would look as cool as the other kids, or as sultry as the women who smoked with long, thin cigarette holders in the movies, so we hunted down her parents' cigarettes and took one out of a pack we found.

We hadn't tried it before, but it didn't matter; we'd both watched our parents light up thousands of times. We walked over to the mirror in my friend's room and she passed me the lighter. I was to go first.

I started picturing how my father and his friends had

gone about lighting up, and with that image in my mind I slowly tucked the cigarette in between my fingers of my right hand and put the cigarette in my mouth. Then I fumbled the lighter in my left hand to spark up a flame and light my first cigarette.

I made my first attempt at inhaling tobacco smoke, which resulted in a "bum puff," where the smoke is let out of the smoker's mouth without being drawn into the lungs. I didn't feel anything, but I had a foul taste of cigarette lingering on my tongue and at the top of my palette. I didn't like the taste, but it didn't matter because everyone else cool did. I also wasn't sure the cigarette had done anything for me, or if I had done it right. Before I could try again, my friend took the lit cigarette from my hand and started to drag on it.

She took in a deep breath and pulled the cigarette out of her mouth. Then her eyes widened and she started coughing profusely, and out came the smoke. We both knew she had just successfully taken her very first drag of tobacco smoke.

"How does it feel?" I asked eagerly as her coughing started to ease up.

She frowned and said, "It's strange; I feel a bit dizzy in my head, and I feel like my feet are really heavy, like stone, sinking into the ground."

She passed the cigarette back to me. "Try again! And remember to breathe in more after you pull the cigarette out!"

I drew back on the cigarette again. This time, I felt a little bit more relaxed than on my first try. Before I sealed my lips, I replayed in my mind how my father and his friends would smoke their cigarettes, how they would breathe in and then pull out the cigarette before that breath was over. This time, I knew exactly how I was going to smoke. I took a deep inhalation and started breathing in. Then I removed the cigarette from my mouth and, without hesitation, I took in more air.

Immediately I felt a strange rush, a gushing into my head, and I started to feel heavy and grounded, but dizzy at the same time. The smoke burned and propelled itself out of my body as I choked and heaved, coughing until there was no more air left in my lungs. My natural instincts were trying to tell me that this was poison, but I went against them, determined to keep going and become a smoker.

My friend once again took the cigarette from my hand and took another puff, coughing a little less, and then I did it again too. We passed the smoke back and forth until the burn had reached the filter. We put the cigarette out in an ashtray and collapsed on to the floor, staring at the ceiling and still coughing. It was a weird feeling, that first cigarette.

It didn't take long before smoking became a habit, a dirty habit that made me feel mature beyond my years when I was still a teenager. Smoking became second nature; I didn't have to replay the way my father smoked anymore. My friends and I started to smoke anywhere and everywhere, and we felt rebellious doing it. We smoked at the bus stop waiting to go to school. We smoked at school in the toilets and down at the sports oval. Once we got home from school, we would hide somewhere down by the creek or in a corner in the park to smoke some more.

Eventually, it didn't matter if I wanted a cigarette or not, I just had to have one! My body dictated when I'd have one. I was no longer able to sleep in because I woke craving nicotine, and wanted to feel the smoke permeate my lungs again. I remember when I was fifteen; I went camping with some friends and smoked a whole packet of cigarettes in one night. All twenty-five cigarettes in eight hours! I became very ill from those cigarettes. I felt sickened and disgusted by how many cigarettes I had just smoked, and how much soot was now clogging up my lungs, but feeling ill that one night didn't stop me from lighting up a cigarette first thing in the morning.

More than fifteen years after that first cigarette I had with my friend, I started trying to quit. I realized smoking wasn't cool anymore. By then, nobody smoked; all the friends who used to smoke with me had stopped. Offices, restaurants, airports, and everywhere else started banning smoking indoors. During the winter months I'd be the only one standing outside in the frigid cold, shivering, desperately sucking in the tobacco smoke, hurriedly getting my nicotine fix despite how uncomfortable every other part of me felt doing it. Every time I smoked, I knew how other people saw me: they thought that I was weak and that I was slowly killing myself with each cigarette. I knew all the harmful effects of smoking, the high risk of emphysema and lung cancer, among other poor health outcomes. I felt guilty about my smoking.

But quitting never worked. I failed each and every time. I'd succumb to a craving and buy a pack and then smoke it all, feeling guilty and bad about myself, and then smoking more to compensate for how I felt, even though smoking never made me feel any better. By then, smoking had stopped making me feel cool, and it had stopped giving me those head rushes that weren't actually a great feeling in the first place.

During the toughest moments of my journey to stop smoking, I've always gone back to that memory of my first cigarette. I remember everything about that first cigarette I shared with my best friend when we were young teenagers: the way the cigarette made me feel, the way I looked in the mirror as I slowly exhaled the white smoke out of my mouth, the way the room spun and the floors sunk after the last puff. I remember thinking that I now belonged with the other cool kids who smoked.

And when I was revisiting that virgin moment, I would always cringe and wish it had never happened. I wished I hadn't conformed to society at the time and buckled to peer pressure. I wished it wasn't so easy to find a cigarette and smoke it. I wished we didn't have role models everywhere who made smoking seem so cool.

Wishing never did anything. Wishing I had never started smoking was never going to help me stop. Instead, it lent the mentality of "Well, since I've started, I might as well keep doing it." And it was the wrong mentality, because stopping smoking can reverse a lot of the harm that earlier smoking has done.

After twenty-seven years of smoking, I finally stopped and am now a non-smoker. If anyone asked me if I wanted a cigarette, I'd now say, "No, I don't smoke." I say it as though I had never smoked in my life, as though I had never struggled with my addiction. This is the mentality that I needed, and that I used in order to stop smoking forever.

I tried quitting many times during my smoking years. The longest period of time I ever managed to quit for was *three* days. And during those attempts, I never felt like I could tell someone I didn't smoke, as I was dying to have a cigarette. Quitting smoking was like a cliff I wasn't ready to jump off, and every effort to stop was just me inching towards the cliff. Each time anyone asked me if I wanted a cigarette, they were pulling me away from the edge and back into the safety and comfort of smoking.

Eventually, I switched paths. I stopped thinking of the cliff and of quitting smoking. I started to think about *stopping* smoking. The cliff disappeared and *stopping* smoking became a journey that wasn't about success or failure, nor fear or worry, and wasn't about that voice in your head that makes you think you won't be able to stop forever. Becoming smoke-free became a continual process. If I succumbed to a craving and had a puff from a cigarette, I could do it without feeling guilty and without having to think that I had failed myself in any way. I simply accepted that it could happen, that it didn't mean I had to go right back to the beginning and inch my way towards a cliff again; I was simply going through my *own* process that I needed to go through to stop. I now wanted to be cool by *not* smoking.

With the right mindset and the right mentality, I have now stopped smoking. The thought of cigarettes no longer stirs up fearful, guilty emotions, nor does it make me deeply ache and crave for tobacco smoke to swim through my lungs, and no longer thinking about those things is the *best* feeling in the world.

Chapter 2

Trials and Tribulations of 'Quitting': How I Finally Stopped'

After smoking up to fifty cigarettes, if not more, every day for sixty years, my father died in January 2013 from cancer that had spread throughout his body. Although smoking might not have been the sole cause of his death, it surely was one of the main contributing factors. He had lung cancer, along with other cancers, when he died.

Some might say my father had a good smoking life for sixty years, but the truth is very different.

Smoking had been negatively impacting his life for a long time before his cancer. Twenty years before my father's death, he was nearly killed by a massive heart attack to which his long-term smoking contributed, and seven years before his death he lost the ability to walk. He developed clogged arteries in his legs, which led to numbness and profuse aching in his legs. But even before he lost his mobility, he had already become a hermit. For a long time he barely left home because it was the only haven left for smoking. Smoking had been banned from too many places so he never went out.

Watching my father suffer and eventually die probably affected my own experiences with smoking. When I smoked, I'd worry about every ache and pain in my body. If my leg hurt, I thought it was from smoking. If I had tenderness or soreness in my throat, I thought it was the smoking. I was constantly feeling anxious or paranoid about when I would become ill with one of the numerous smoking-related diseases.

Smoking kills – that's what they tell us.

According to the World Health Organization,[1] tobacco kills up to *six million people each year*. Worldwide, tobacco *kills one person every six seconds and accounts for one in ten adult deaths*. Up to half of all current users will eventually die of a tobacco-related disease. And smoking doesn't affect only your mouth, throat, lungs, and heart – it affects nearly every single organ in the body.

But it wasn't death or the fear of dying that led me to stop smoking. I wasn't scared of dying – I was scared of living. I was terrified of living with the consequences of smoking, with all the ailments I would eventually get as a direct result of my habit. Smoking kills, yes, but it usually

---

[1] *"World Health Organization Media Centre Fact Sheet N°339: Tobacco," World Health Organization, last modified July 2013, accessed September 3, 2013. http://www.who.int/mediacentre/factsheets/fs339/en/.*

kills you slowly, gradually, and the slow death of your body, be it because your lungs slowly stop working and you start having difficulties breathing on your own, or because you get cancer, is bound to be an unpleasant experience. Whichever way smoking might eventually kill me, I simply didn't want that for myself. I wanted to stop smoking so I could live both longer and healthier. I wanted to breathe. Breathing is one of the things in life that we *have* to do, or we *will* die. Breathing became more important to me than smoking.

I knew I had to stop so I could live free from this fear. That was my main reason for quitting, but everyone's reason could be different; yours could be that you want to run without wheezing, or are planning on becoming pregnant, or don't want to expose your kids to secondhand smoke. Whatever your reason, there is always a way to stop smoking and it is *never* too late.

After years and decades of trying, I finally accomplished what I had wanted. I finally stopped smoking for good, and I want to share my experience as a way of taking you and other struggling smokers down this path as well.

Stopping smoking is about persistence. It is probably one

of the toughest challenges I've had to overcome in my life.

I managed to stop smoking cigarettes because I persevered and had my coach to encourage me. It's not because of some quit date I set, or some helpline I called, or some nicotine patch I used. I've heard some people say, "You know, one day I woke up, and I just didn't want to smoke anymore, and that was the end of it." That also wasn't the case for me. I thought I loved smoking and, most of all, my body and mind were completely addicted to both the act of inhaling cigarette smoke and the nicotine.

During my attempts to stop smoking I tried every method in the book. One of the most commonly used methods is a "quit date," in which you mark down a date on which you commit to quitting and never smoke again after that. Over fifteen years of attempting to quit I tried the "quit date" method about twelve times and it never worked. In retrospect, I think it's because setting a quit date was just too terrifying. The thought of never being able to smoke again didn't sit well with me, and at the first sign of a craving I'd buckle and resolve that I just couldn't quit forever.

After smoking a pack a day, and thinking that I enjoyed it, it was fairly hard to fathom not smoking ever again. So then I would buy a pack of cigarettes, and smoke all of it. I'd feel guilty about doing it, and I'd feel like I'd let myself down, yet again, and that would propel me to smoke even more as a form of comfort.

Besides setting a quit date, I tried quitting cold turkey. I also tried other countless remedies that never lasted more than three hours. I don't want to name these methods, as I don't want to taint them for my readers if they haven't tried them. All smoking cessation aid devices are meant to target your addiction, to suppress your cravings, or to reduce nicotine withdrawal symptoms, but they didn't work for me. And I'm not alone on this. I do, however, know other people who have succeeded using these methods.

The reason I think they don't work for some people, is because using them alone without the proper mindset will not make you stop. They are merely intended to help reduce your cravings and to suppress nicotine withdrawal symptoms. The rest of the work is up to you.

I learned this the hard way, after spending many hours and lots of money trying out all the different therapies out there. I sometimes feel so mad that I listened to the "experts" and all it did was make me smoke more each time I failed. It wasn't until I found my own approach to stopping smoking that I actually got the results I wanted.

As most smokers know, we are addicted to and dependent upon nicotine, and for that reason and that reason only we smoke cigarettes.

Here's a brief outline to how I stopped; each step will be discussed in greater detail in later chapters:

1. **Change the Thinking** – This was the most important step. My biggest mistake with my previous attempts to "quit" was thinking that if I had just *one* cigarette that I had failed and was a full-time smoker once again. What I learned, however, is that it is completely okay if I did have that *one* cigarette. It just meant that I had to keep *persevering*.

2. **Everyone is Different** – It was important for me to realize that just because some people can stop by going cold turkey or stick to a quit date doesn't mean that everyone can do it those ways. We are all different and we will all have our own methods and time

frames that enable us to stop forever.

3. **Cutting Down** – I weaned myself off cigarettes by cutting down in increments of five cigarettes every couple of weeks and gradually arrived at zero per day. If you smoke twenty-five cigarettes per day now, try cutting out five per day, then another five per day after two weeks. If you continued this pattern, you could be down to smoking just five cigarettes per day after only two months. Imagine that: you have been trying to stop for decades and now you are having just five cigarettes per day and it only took you two months. After smoking five per day, you could eventually go to zero per day. **Don't idolize the cigarettes you are having**. Cigarettes are not your friend. They never were and never will be. If you have cut down and are only smoking a few cigarettes per day, don't look at them with admiration, look at them with disdain. They are the reason you are in this situation in the first place.

4. **Personal Coach** – I engaged the services of a personal coach. Michael made me understand that my mind was in survival mode and wanted me to smoke.

5. **Practice Stopping** – Once you to get to zero ciga-rettes per day, you may relapse and have one or two (just like I did). If this happens, please do not despair. Get back on track and practice some more. Practice makes perfect and it is what we have to do to stop smoking. We have to learn how to become non-smokers again, just like we had to learn to smoke in the first place. Eventually, you'll stop thinking about smoking entirely, just as I did.

6. **Break Habits** – I broke old habits each day. For exam-ple, instead of smoking in my smoking area, I smoked in a different place that I don't usually frequent.

7. **Learn More about Smoking** – I got to know the facts about smoking in detail so I knew exactly what I was doing to my body.

8. **Come Up with Strategies** – I came up with thoughts and distractions that would help turn me off smok-ing. For example, imagine spraying fly spray and in-haling it; that is essentially what you're doing when you inhale cigarette smoke.

9. **Develop a Reward System** – Give yourself a reward

for every day you don't smoke. Come up with a reward plan ahead of time so you have something to look forward to as a distraction when you have your next craving. Save your cigarette money and go buy that thing you've been wanting; at fifteen dollars a pack, the savings will soon add up. You deserve it – reward all of your small victories!

10. **Instead of Calling It a Goal, Call It a "Want"** My *want* is to smoke five fewer cigarettes; my *want* is to smoke ten fewer cigarettes; I eventually *want* to not smoke at all.

With my method of stopping, I never set a quit date. Nobody needs that added pressure and stress. Stopping is challenging enough on its own. If you didn't have a cigarette for two days, but then had one after that, you did a *great* job because you stopped for two whole days. That might be twenty, thirty, forty fewer cigarettes – just keep going. If you had stopped for a month, that is nine hundred fewer cigarettes. *Anybody* can stop smoking at any time they choose. Those who say they can't stop smoking just *won't* stop smoking. So choose to stop, choose to let yourself cut down slowly, day by day. Let your mind and your body gradually get used to the idea that you will not be smoking at all one day in the near future. You are not giving up anything when you stop smoking but you are gaining *everything*!

Once you've got the hang of stopping, if you are still finding yourself struggling, get some extra help. Don't just do it alone.

After I hadn't had a cigarette for about four months, I did feel like I needed some extra help. I went to see a psychiatrist and he gave me the best advice I can give anybody for anything they are trying to accomplish in their life: *'take it one day at a time'*. Don't worry about six months down the track; worry about *today*. He also taught me that when you get the feeling that you need a cigarette, just accept that feeling and acknowledge it instead of trying to fight it. Tell yourself, "Okay, I understand the feeling. It's there but it doesn't mean I have to have a cigarette." It was great advice because I'd never really thought about it that way. I always fought the feeling and made myself angry, which didn't help.

If you take anything away from my experience, it's that you must not think of this as *"quitting"* smoking. It's *"stopping"* smoking. The difference is subtle and nuanced, but changing your thinking to use this one simple verb can change your entire experience, like it did for me.

To quit means to give up smoking forever, and to never turn back. That's daunting, and the thought of that was never conducive to actually quitting for me. Just because you relapse and have three or four cigarettes, after having had none for a couple weeks, doesn't mean that you are a smoker again. It doesn't mean that you have to revert back to your old self and smoke full-time. *It's about practicing stopping.* This is what I did for the first three months of my final attempt to stop for good. I would have about three or four cigarettes a day and then I would go to zero for a couple of weeks. Then I'd have one and then stop again. And then I'd go for three weeks without one, and then have a couple, and so on and so forth. It took me about four months to finish my practice, until I had stopped smoking enough times that it became my life to not smoke.

Not smoking has become second nature to me.

I don't even know the official date I stopped, and that's the point – it just happened! I didn't know on the day I was having my last cigarette. But I do remember having it. That last cigarette was like my first: it tasted disgusting and it choked me.

It was funny, but I had always wanted go back and to talk to that teenager, to tell her before she had that first cigarette that she would regret it, that she would rue that day she started, that she should follow her first instinct and stop smoking that foul tasting cigarette. Well it took twenty-seven years but I got that chance, even though it was her last cigarette, not her first!

Chapter 3

Breaking the Habits

To stop smoking is to break a habit. If you've ever tried to break any habit, like having a beer or a glass of wine after you get home from work, or chewing your nails, you know it's challenging. But we break habits all the time, whether it's changing a commute route to work, driving a different car, or using a new remote for the television. Some habits are easier to break than others, but none are impossible to break. Habits are norms, the way we learn to do things over time. It's the same when we try to break or unlearn a habit; it happens gradually over time. When it comes to smoking, you have to be prepared for this challenge in order to succeed. You sometimes have to gradually unlearn a habit.

Breaking the habit of smoking might actually be simpler than you think, the reason being that it's easy to identify other habits that are connected with smoking. Smoking isn't as omnipresent as other habits, largely because there are many occasions and situations in which you can't smoke – unlike biting your nails, for instance. So, the first step to breaking the habit is to identify the routines associated with smoking. These could include having a cigarette with coffee in the morning, or having one after dinner. Once you've recognized these associations, you can plan strategies for breaking them.

There is no singular way to do this. For example, you might want to stop drinking coffee at home so you don't have that cigarette. You might wait until you get to your office, or an indoor café, to have a coffee; this way you don't have the luxury of smoking. Each person has to come up with his or her own strategy, and when one strategy fails to break the association then a new strategy is called for. As the saying goes, *"the definition of madness is doing the same thing over and over again and expecting a different result each time,"* so be creative, change the strategy, and remove the association.

When you get to the point where you're cutting down on cigarettes, try not to have them at the same time each day. If you're only having two a day, for example, don't always have one in the morning and one before you go to bed. That will just create a new association, or reinforce an existing one, and won't help to break the habit. So be conscious of these routines and try not to repeat them from day to day. For example, have a cigarette in the morning one day, and have one in the afternoon the next. Have a cigarette after work one day, but not the next. Don't form new habits or associations. While cutting down on cigarettes, don't smoke at your favorite time or place anymore. By this I mean the _one_ time when smoking gives you the most satisfaction. Whichever cigarettes you enjoy the most, cut them out of your life forever. I cut my morning cigarettes out first because they were my favorite.

Like the first time you smoked, stopping smoking is a conscious decision. It's about discovering and acknowledging your cravings, habits, and routines. It's about brainstorming, trial and error, and finding the right strategy for the problem.

Smoking is associated with more than specific activities, like talking or drinking. I smoked for different emotions. When I was sad, I'd smoke. When I felt defeated, I'd smoke. I'd smoke when I was lonely, or when I was excited. These are all associations that need to be disrupted. You have to come up with strategies or replacements. If you're tired and need to re-energize, don't have that cigarette. Go for a short walk to get a coffee, or maybe even go for a short, brisk jog. Remember, one day at a time.

Remember, there just isn't a one-size-fits-all strategy

for breaking the habit.

Don't rush this part. The idea is to slowly cut down and to not place too much stress on yourself while stopping, to avoid triggering a relapse. Take it slowly and change each smoking habit one at a time; don't try to break them all at once.

The first habit I broke was smoking in my usual area. If there is a place where you always smoke, like your porch, don't go to it. I closed the door and the curtain so I couldn't even see it, so I wouldn't be reminded of it. You'll still think of it, but at least it's not as obvious. **Never smoke in that area again**. Smoke somewhere that is different and that you can't see so you are not constantly reminded of smoking. If you smoke inside, **stop and never smoke inside again**. Make that your golden rule. Each time you feel like smoking, take your cigarette outside; this alone should help cut down the number of cigarettes you have each day. Then you can go from there, and start to reduce the number of trips outside also.

We all have and need rules in our life. Some of our rules may prohibit us from eating particular foods or drinking sugary drinks, or limit how much we spend on clothing.

There is nothing wrong with having smoking rules as well. We ought to have them.

One of the first habits I broke was smoking while talking on the phone. This was a pretty easy one to start with for me. Instead of grabbing for my packet as soon as the phone rang, I'd pick up the phone and concentrate on the conversation. This soon became the norm for me and I broke the habit completely within a week. The following week, I broke the habit of smoking while in the car. If I was craving a cigarette I'd just crank up the music and sing really loudly instead. The week after that, I tried not to smoke right away after dinner; instead, I'd give myself half an hour or so before I was allowed to have a cigarette. Eventually, I would just forget about that after-dinner cigarette because I'd start doing something else and become distracted. From my own experience, it doesn't take long to break old habits. Try breaking one per week.

Change your environment. I remember having a really bad day and not wanting to go home. I told my husband that the house reminded me too much of smoking. When I got home he had rearranged the furniture in the lounge room for me – a small change, but it did help. Just having my favorite chair positioned in a different place altered my usual path for passing through the room and going outside to smoke.

Have something to look forward to in the morning or whenever you miss cigarettes the most. My most missed cigarettes were the morning ones. My mornings used to consist of getting up, putting the kettle on, going outside to have my first cigarette, and then having a cup of tea. I am embarrassed to say this, but I used to have at least three cigarettes over the span of an hour with a cup of tea *every* morning. In order to break this habit, I stopped going outside for my tea. Instead, I recorded all of my favorite TV programs the night before so I had something to look forward to in the morning, and I would have a cup of tea while watching those shows. Now I don't even need to turn on the TV, and I can sit in my "ex-smoking room" and drink tea without a problem. I have broken that association. Try it – you'll be surprised.

If your worst time is in the evening after dinner or just before you go to bed, find a different activity to do. The activity may not seem enjoyable at first, but it will soon become a new habit, replacing the old one. If you have your worst cigarette cravings before you go to bed, get hold of a really good book or find a great TV show to enjoy in bed without a cigarette. There are hundreds of things we can do instead, but in the past we have just chosen to smoke.

As with smoking at different times of the day, try to smoke in different places so that no single place becomes associated with smoking. When I was stopping, I would never smoke my rare cigarettes in my usual place. Instead, I would go for a walk and smoke somewhere totally foreign to me, so that it didn't feel like I was slipping back into my old habit again. As long as I could still smoke, I was happy to smoke anywhere. I will say this again: if you have an outdoor area that you usually smoke in, stop now! Never smoke there again. Remove all ashtrays. Buy a new pot plant or a table runner and make this area as pleasant and cheerful as possible without cigarettes.

I also bought different brands of cigarette. Instead of buying my favorite cigarettes, I would buy ones that I didn't really like. This helped immensely because I wasn't experiencing my usual taste. If you don't like a particular brand or strength of cigarette, buy them instead; they will soon turn you off smoking. Make sure you don't buy a brand that you totally dislike as you may just go back to buying your favorite cigarettes. Also, try to switch brands often; you don't want to become tolerant of and familiar with a particular taste.

The key here is that you want to break all your old smoking habits without introducing new ones. You have to try and be vigilant with each cigarette you have. Take note of when you had it, where you had it, who you might have had it with, and try not to repeat yourself. Keep a log of your habits and routines if that's helpful.

After you have gone about destroying all your old habits, there are some other neat ways to support your continued efforts to stop smoking. If you have a smartphone, download some smoking cessation apps. There are all sorts of cool and *free* apps for your phone now. Some tell you how much money you are saving as you progress through your journey, and others tell you how much tar has *not* entered your lungs and other vital statistics about your health. These apps could be fun, informative, and helpful in recognizing what you have achieved as you cut down and eventually stop. Who wouldn't like to know they saved four hundred dollars in a month because they smoked thirty fewer packs?

In addition to those apps that help you tally up all your gains since cutting down or stopping, you could even start a DIY project to help visualize them. For example, you could have a jar for the money that you would have spent on cigarettes but didn't. If you go from smoking a pack a day to a pack a week, place the amount a pack is worth into your jar for each day you don't buy one. If you don't have cash, instead of going to buy a pack of cigarettes on your credit or debit card you can go to the bank and take out the equivalent amount of money and save that in your jar. If you are the artistic type, you can probably dream up even better ways to help visualize the greatness of your efforts. For example, you might want to buy a new motor-bike. You could have a picture of that motorbike and high-light pieces that you could have already paid for. You might already own the front tire and the fuel tank.

In conclusion, try to come up with as many strategies as you can to break your smoking habits. Visualize your efforts by seeing the money pile up in your jar, change your routines, switch the times and places of your cigarettes. Your strategies can be as simple as taking deep breaths for two minutes, mimicking the length in time you would spend inhaling and exhaling tobacco smoke, or maybe putting something in between your fingers that feels like a cigarette (like a straw or a pen) and taking deep breaths from it.

But whatever you do, don't try to break your smoking habits by replacing the cigarettes with food. You don't want your mind or body to wrongly think that stopping smoking is making you gain weight. If you do end up gaining weight, you may use this as an excuse to start smoking full-time again.

I smoked for twenty-seven years and it only took me a couple of months to break all my smoking habits, and from there stopping became much easier. I think that's a pretty fair deal. Once you break your old habits, you are now *in control*. I love that it's me, not the nicotine, who's in control of my body and mind. If we let the nicotine control us, it will also inevitably decide our deaths as well – do you really want that?

Behind the smoking habit there is just an addiction. If you can cut down your smoking and ease out the addiction then breaking the habit could be more easily done.

One last set of habits to consider is the people around you who smoke and who you might frequently smoke together with. I was very fortunate in that I did not have many smokers around me when I was stopping, which helped immensely. If many of your friends, colleagues, or family members smoke, it will be a bigger challenge to break the social habit of smoking. No matter how difficult it might be, you have to try and break this habit. If you enjoy competition, try starting one with your friends or colleagues who smoke to see who can cut down the most and have a prize for the winner. Why not take the money you're all saving and place it in a pool, winner-take-all?

Get in the habit of looking at smoking environments as places you don't want to be in – look carefully. If you are at a hotel, airport, or restaurant and there is a designated smoking area, pay attention to what really goes on in there. There are dirty ashtrays everywhere, there are usually a few butts still burning away in a rubbish bin, the room is hazy and smells of stale smoke, and people are packed inside of it, smoking as quickly as they can so they can get out of there. Once you stop smoking, you never need to ever, ever go into a Designated Outdoor Smoking Area (DOSA), or a dingy designated smoking room inside an airport ever again. And thank heavens for that.

If your partner smokes, ask him or her to support your efforts to stop by not smoking around you. They could smoke in another room, or go around the corner so that they're not within your sight. If they can't make that small effort for you, then they are not being supportive during what might be one of your most trying times.

The same applies to other friends, co-workers, and family members. Either you can try and remove yourself from them when they are about to smoke, or you can kindly ask them not to smoke around you. Be wary of anyone who might offer you a cigarette even though they know you are stopping. It could be that they want you to smoke with them so they can feel better about themselves. If you are around smokers and you are not smoking, be proud that you are a stronger person than the person smoking and you know it.

Chapter 4

The Good Stuff You Should Know about Stopping

The majority of active smokers want to stop at some point – maybe not now, but at a later date. In the United States, about seventy percent of all smokers want to quit and forty percent will try this year.[2] Only seven percent of smokers succeed at quitting their first time,[3] and about four to five percent of smokers who try to quit in any given year will succeed in stopping smoking permanently.[4] These numbers seem daunting, but what is more encouraging is that nearly forty to fifty percent of smokers will eventually succeed in quitting, after trying many times over.[5] Furthermore, studies have shown that if you can stop for three months – three months is all it takes – then you most likely will never smoke again. This was the case with me.

I am one of those who have succeeded after numerous repeated attempts.

---

[2] "Quitting Smoking Statistics," Statistic Brain, last modified July 28, 2013, accessed September 4, 2013, http://www.statisticbrain.com/quitting-smoking-statistics/.

[3] Ibid.
[4] Dunston, Ashlee, Kicking Butts in the Twenty-First Century: What Modern Science Has Learned about Smoking Cessation (New York: American Council on Science and Health, 2003), http://acsh.org/2003/08/kicking-butts-in-the-twenty-first-century/.
[5] Ibid.

As a smoker thinking of or trying to stop, scare tactics never worked for me. And that's why this book isn't about scare tactics. I don't need someone to tell me I'm going to die from smoking, or that I'm filling my lungs with tar with each drag from a cigarette. Trying to motivate me to stop smoking by instilling fear only makes me less motivated to stop.

For many who are trying to quit, especially heavier smokers, these tactics instill a sense of shame. They make people feel inferior to or lesser than others when it comes to their smoking habits. Instead of this encouraging them to explore avenues to help them, this demotivates people's want to stop smoking (as a means of dealing with the shame), and often discourages people from attempting to engage in discussions with friends, doctors, or others, out of fear that they would be shamed for continuing the practice.

These tactics are also ineffective because they are trying to expose people to the long-term effects of smoking, which are not yet tangible to them. Most people live day-to-day; we live for the short-term and not for tomorrow. When popularized mottos in society include "carpe diem" and "live for today" it's pretty difficult to make decisions in relation to what might happen ten, twenty, forty, or even fifty years from now.

Having said all that, even though it's hard to think too far into the future, it is good to remind yourself while you're stopping that fifty percent of active smokers will die from smoking-related causes. Thinking, *"I'm going to die anyway; I might as well smoke,"* is probably not the wisest behavior, because dying from other causes is likely going to be much more pleasant than dying from smoking-related illness. Nobody wants to suffer before they die, nobody wants to be hooked up to an oxygen tank or have a lung removed while they wait for their death, and nobody wants to have emphysema and always feel short of breath.

But again, knowing the harms of smoking isn't enough. Scare tactics don't necessarily help smokers to reach the decision to stop, but they can provide another reason to continue not smoking.

Deciding to stop has to stem from your own desire. Never pressure yourself to stop because of scare tactics or because of societal and peer pressure. Attempting to stop because of external forces and reasons is unlikely to result in success. You have to take the time to explore your own addiction and habits, and recognize your reasons for smoking and for stopping. If your peers or family start pressuring you, or criticizing and shaming you for having a smoke while you are trying to stop, let them know that you are taking this at your own pace and according to your own will. It is important to be mindful of what others might and will say while you are trying to stop, and to remind yourself that this decision is yours alone to make. If you have a craving and decide to have a cigarette, that is your own choice and you should recognize that you're still stopping, and that this one cigarette doesn't mark a complete relapse.

Given the importance of self-awareness and your own will to stopping smoking, it is helpful to learn about the benefits. Knowing these could help you formulate strong, resilient reasoning for stopping.

Before you learn about the benefits of stopping, it is good to know what you are inhaling into your body when you smoke a cigarette. That way you know exactly what's *not* entering your body anymore when you stop, or even if you just cut down.

There are more than 7,000 chemicals in tobacco smoke and at least 250 are harmful, including hydrogen cyanide and ammonia.[6] Of these harmful chemicals, at least 69 are cancer-causing, including arsenic, benzene, beryllium (a toxic metal), cadmium (another toxic metal), and polonium-210 (a radioactive element). Suffice it to say, tobacco smoke is more than just nicotine and tar. It can cause all sorts of illnesses and cancers, including cancers of the lung, esophagus, cervix, mouth, throat, kidney, pancreas, bladder, and stomach, as well as acute myeloid leukemia. Smoking is a leading cause of cancer and cancer-related death.

Without getting into too many details, here are some of the harms of smoking[7]:

- Increased risk of cancer (the risk of lung cancer increases by thirteen to twenty-three times)

- Increased risk of heart disease (by two to four times), stroke (by two to four times), and aortic aneurysm (which is a bulge in or dilation of your aorta, which

---

[6] *"Harms of Smoking and Health Benefits of Quitting," National Cancer Institute, last modified January 12, 2011, accessed 3 September 3, 2013,* http://www.cancer.gov/cancertopics/factsheet/Tobacco/cessation.
[7] *Ibid.*

originates from your heart and is the largest artery in your body, that can kill you if it ruptures)

- Risk of chronic obstructive pulmonary disease (COPD), which can take the form of chronic bronchitis (chronic coughing with mucus, often accompanied by occasional chest pains) or emphysema (in which your lung tissues deteriorate and lose elasticity, making breathing difficult and causing a chronic shortness of breath as well as coughing and mucus)

- Risk of narrowing of the blood vessels, which can lead to obstruction of large arteries in the legs and arms, and cause pain, tissue loss, and, in prolonged cases, gangrene

- Risk of asthma

- Risk of cataracts (which affect the eye and can lead to blindness)

- Greater risk of erectile dysfunction

- Increased risk of infertility, preterm delivery, stillbirth, low birth weight, and sudden infant death syndrome

Basically, one of the benefits of stopping smoking is a reduction of all risks, and after stopping for decades your risk of maladies could be close or equal to a non-smoker's. You're never too old and it's never too late to stop; you will always benefit, and within days and weeks you will be able to feel the positive differences: reduction in coughing and sputum, less wheezing when you exercise, better blood circulation, less anxiety, more energy, an improved immune system and therefore less illness, and just an overall improvement in health and wellbeing. Your sense of smell and taste will also increase, your teeth won't be all stained, you won't smell of stale smoke anymore, and your skin will look better. Not to mention, if you stop smoking – be it for a few days or years – you can be proud of what you have accomplished and feel good about that, and you will have saved a lot of money by not buying cigarettes.

Not smoking means you can stay healthy into an older age – without having to live with emphysema, have your tongue cut out, or have difficulty breathing for the rest of your days.

If you are still smoking in ten years, what will it be

like? There will probably be nowhere left in public where you can smoke – as it is, smoking has become more frowned upon and less acceptable in public. You probably won't even be able to smoke on your own property because the smoke will go into someone else's yard. You won't be able to smoke on balconies because the smoke will go into other people's units. You will look terrible. A packet of cigarettes will probably cost about three hundred dollars. They may even be illegal. Is this all worth it? Besides fulfilling a habit, did the last cigarette you have actually make a positive difference for you?

Every cigarette you 'don't' have is doing you good. And in case you've never seen this before, here's a list outlining what you can look forward to at different points in time after you've stopped smoking[8]:

- After twenty minutes:
  - Blood pressure and pulse return to normal.

---

[8] *This list is adapted from the following sources:*
"Stop Smoking Recovery Timetable," WhyQuit.com, last modified February 13, 2013, http://whyquit.com/whyquit/a_benefits_time_table.html.
"Heart and Vascular Health & Prevention: Smoking and Heart Disease," Cleveland Clinic,
http://my.clevelandclinic.org/heart/prevention/smoking/smoking_hrtds.aspx.

- o The temperature of your hands and feet returns to normal.
- After eight to twelve hours:
  - o The carbon monoxide and oxygen levels in your blood return to normal.
- After twenty-four hours:
  - o The risk of heart attack decreases and your anxiety levels due to nicotine withdrawal peak, and will decrease from here on out.
- After forty-eight hours:
  - o Nerve endings begin to adjust to the absence of nicotine and your sense of taste and smell improves.
  - o Anger and irritation associated with stopping smoking have peaked and start to fall.
  - o Smoker's cough is nearly non-existent.
- After seventy-two hours:
  - o Your craving episodes peak around now and will start to decrease from here on out.
  - o Your body is now *100% nicotine-free* and your breathing starts to become easier.
- After five to eight days:

- o The number of cue-induced cravings average around three per day, and each lasts no longer than three minutes. (Just keep this in mind next time you have a craving: know that in a matter of minutes your mind will have moved on to something else.)
- After two weeks to three months:

  - o Anger, anxiety, difficulty concentrating, restlessness, fatigue, insomnia and depression associated with stopping smoking have now passed.
  - o Your circulation and lung function start to improve, your risk of heart attacks has started to drop, you feel more energetic, and you can exercise easily.
- After one year:

  - o Your risk of heart disease is now half that of a current smoker.
- After five to fifteen years:

  - o Your risk of stroke is now the same as that of someone who has never smoked.
- After ten years:

  - o Your risk of dying from lung cancer is almost the

same as that of someone who has never smoked.

- o Your risk of cancers of the mouth, larynx, esophagus, bladder, kidney, and pancreas has also decreased.
- After fifteen years:

  - o Your risk of heart disease is the same as someone who has never smoked.

Okay, thinking ahead in "years" – one year, five years, ten years, fifteen years – may seem daunting and terrifying. But don't be scared by it. As mentioned before, statistics have shown that you just have to hold out for three months. If you can stop smoking for three months, you will have a very good chance of succeeding. And by then, you won't even have to think about stopping anymore – you will simply *be* a non-smoker.

If you have decided to stop smoking, and have succeeded in stopping for a day, a week, or a month, or more, and someone asks you whether you smoke, try this: tell them you are a non-smoker. Be brave and proud – start thinking of yourself as someone who doesn't smoke, who doesn't want to or need to.

Remember, it's just *three* minutes of cravings *three*

times a day for *three* months and you're set for the rest of your life. That's all it is. And don't forget to think of all the reasons you have and had thought of when you decided to stop.

Remember the rule of three!

Can you find something to occupy your mind for three minutes? Check your email, take a short walk around the block, make a coffee, grab a drink of water from the water fountain on another floor at work (using the stairs of course), or have a quick chat with a coworker. Pretty soon the cravings pass and you're on your way again.

Chapter 5

Thoughts for When You're Stopping

Despite the strategies you've come up with to break the habit and the reasons you've come up with to stop smoking, the cravings will come. They could come about naturally as a result of associations with emotions and other activities, or they could surface because you smell cigarette smoke while strolling through a park, or because you see smokers hanging around outside of a bar. Cravings come and go, but even if a craving episode lasts less than three minutes, each feels like eternity.

Everyone needs a coping mechanism to ease them through a craving episode. You have to find a distraction (physical or mental) that could make the three minutes actually feel like seconds or even less. But at the exact moment of a craving, it can be pretty hard to think up a reason why you shouldn't satisfy your craving. So have a distraction ready to go at anytime. Always remember to accept the craving; don't try to ignore or fight it, just understand what it is.

When you've decided to stop smoking and have started cutting down, come up with a list of thoughts that might help fend off having a cigarette during a craving attack. Remember, it is important to try and disrupt rhythm and routine when you're cutting down. So if you had a cigarette after dinner yesterday, and you want one right after dinner today, tell yourself: "just thirty more minutes and I can have one." You could also try leaving your cigarettes at home when you go out so that when you have a craving you can calm yourself with the fact that you can have one (thirty minutes) after you get home.

When you are stopping and a craving comes up, think of something that will make you not want the cigarette. Staring at the warning images on cigarette packages probably won't do the trick; instead, try taking a deep breath. Take note of how good a deep breath feels. Inhale deeply, right down into your lungs, and exhale long. Count your breaths. Then, imagine what it would be like if that feeling of breathing was taken away from you. If that doesn't work for you, here are some more thoughts I've used to suppress my cravings when they've come along in the past:

Realize we have been brainwashed about the benefits of smoking. We all know that smoking tobacco is extremely harmful to us, but we still do it. Why is this? When we were growing up we were bombarded with messages that cigarettes help us relax, concentrate and handle stress. We form the belief that cigarettes are special, precious things and that we are somehow incomplete without them.

Do you suppose that if we had never started smoking in the first place we would need nicotine to carry out our daily lives?

Smokers are paying tobacco companies to kill them in the most horrible way. If you are thinking of stopping, it's probably because you are trying to become healthier. If so, you are probably making healthier choices in other aspects of your life. Maybe you're exercising more, or maybe you're eating better. When you smoke, not only are you paying a corporate giant to shorten your life, but you are also paying them to reverse all the health gains you've made from your other healthy choices (which you probably also had to pay for – living a healthy lifestyle often comes with a price tag). Or imagine this: if water companies were putting poisons into your water, which would slowly but surely kill you, you would be *outraged* and would *definitely* stop drinking that water. So why don't you want to breathe clean air, and why would you pay a company to give you toxins to kill you?

Instead of giving all of that money to tobacco companies, wouldn't you rather spend it on yourself or your loved ones? How long has it been since you took your kids on a holiday?

Don't idolize cigarettes. Cigarettes are not your friend. They never were and never will be. If you have cut down and are only smoking a few per day, don't look at them with admiration, look at them with disdain. They are the reason you are in this situation in the first place.

Imagine smoking a cigarette with a wet butt. Imagine if the butt of the cigarette was soaking wet and you smoked it. All of the tar and chemicals would be mixed with the water and end up in your mouth.

Put cigarette butts in a jar of water and imagine that you had to drink the water. Think of what you would be putting in your mouth, including hydrogen cyanide, ammonia, arsenic, cadmium (another toxic metal), and polonium-210. If you can just imagine drinking your cigarette instead of smoking it, you'll probably not want it anymore. It's the nasty thought that counts.

Look away. This is simple enough. If you're watching someone smoke, or you can smell the smoke, that craving is probably going to last. Get out of there. If you can't get out of there, which may sometimes be the case, then *look closely.* Don't look closely in the sense of looking at the person smoking and imagining how good it would feel if it was you. No, look closely and just try to imagine yourself looking through an x-ray machine at the black tar and all the toxic stuff that is going into the person's lungs, slowly clogging them up and leaving them short of breath and chronically phlegmy. Now take a deep breath. Maybe you don't want that cigarette anymore because your breath felt better than the black tar chemical smoke.

Take deep breaths. Taking deep breaths can be enough to satisfy your craving — especially if you use a prop like a straw or something to inhale through. Just think to yourself that you are doing exactly the same thing as you would be if you were smoking, except clean air is going into your lungs and not toxic waste. Close your eyes, breathe in very deeply, and hold your breath for a count of three, then exhale for a count of three. Let your body relax and lose the tension built-up from craving and wanting nicotine and cigarettes.

Take it one day at a time. Remind yourself to take it

one day at a time, one craving at a time. Don't start to panic. Don't think about the next craving you will have or all the cravings you might have in the future. Just think of right now. This craving isn't going to last for more than three minutes. It won't last forever.

Recall the risk of disease and death. If the prospect of death, or one of the many diseases that could render you generally breathless and immobile, or even bedridden (like a stroke for example), scares you, hold that thought. As smokers, we often say *"we know what we are doing to ourselves when we smoke."* But we don't always. Think about what it would be like to have lung cancer or emphysema. Think about life without your tongue or your mouth and jaw. Think about having no teeth or getting gangrene in your feet. Think about having to rely on others to help you get around and help you go to the toilet. Think about how many needles you will need to get if you have to go to hospital. External scare tactics might not be effective, but internal scare tactics might actually do the trick.

Recognize that it's embarrassing when you wheeze. Maybe you feel embarrassed sometimes when you become short of breath just from walking up a flight of stairs. Know that the shortness of breath and wheezing isn't you – that's the smoking. If you stop, you won't have to be embarrassed about your wheezing or your lack of athleticism anymore.

Google images of smoking effects. If you have a smartphone on hand, or you're near a computer, you might as well Google some images of the effects of smoking. Those will surely make you not want a cigarette right now.

Think of the benefits. Recall all the benefits of not smoking. Your heart works better, you're less likely to suffer a stroke, you're breathing better, and you're more energetic. You've also probably overcome several or numerous cravings already. Why would you waste all those efforts now? If you do, you're going to have to start again. Remember, the craving you are having right now is weaker than the craving you had the last time, and the one before that. You've made it this far. You just have this one craving to overcome and your risk of developing all those different diseases will have dropped, and your overall health and appearance will have improved.

You're saving money. A craving hits and you don't

have cigarettes because you haven't needed or wanted or had one in a while. You either have to ask someone for one, or you have to spend fifteen dollars on a new pack you will regret buying. How could you otherwise spend that fifteen dollars? Then imagine if you continued to smoke. Ten years from now, a pack of cigarettes might be two, or maybe even three hundred dollars. Who knows? You don't want to be caught in that situation. Here is a good question: how much would you be willing to pay for a packet of cigarettes tomorrow? What if you woke up and cigarettes were two hundred dollars per pack? Would you pay that? I bet you would buy one pack and smoke one or two cigarettes per day, and then you wouldn't smoke any more.

You don't actually want that cigarette. Just try to convince yourself that you are a non-smoker. You actually don't want that cigarette and *your body doesn't actually need it*. You don't need that "one last" cigarette or puff. You really don't. You haven't had one in a while and you're doing just fine. That puff won't do you any good. It won't help with any future cravings; in fact, it'll just make the next one worse. That puff will set you back. The nicotine levels in your body will go back up. Your blood circulation will drop. You'll lose the benefits you will have made in improving your sense of taste and smell. You are a non-smoker and smoking is no longer a habit. You don't want that cigarette.

Supposing you haven't had a cigarette in three years. Don't think of having just *one* cigarette – what's the use? I know you feel healthier now and you think you could handle having the occasional cigarette because you have stopped in the past. You're curious to see what a cigarette would feel like again. Even though you might assure yourself that it won't make you a smoker again, and that you've stopped for three years, and that you won't start again, don't have that *one* cigarette. A cigarette is a cigarette is a cigarette. One puff and you'll reverse a lot of the gains you've made over the three years. If you want to be a non-smoker, why would you smoke any amount of cigarettes? It doesn't make sense.

Don't only think distracting thoughts; do something distracting. For example, go wash your hair or take a shower. Or you can brush your teeth and enjoy the fresh feeling in your mouth. I have a friend who did star jumps *every time* he had a craving. It didn't have to be for long, just long enough to quicken his breath and increase his heart rate. He'd even do it when he was at work (he is a bartender). Think of it as a prolonged toilet break. Or even better, think of it as the same amount of time as a smoking break (five minutes or more). If you can take five minutes off whatever it is you're doing to have a smoke break, you can take that same amount of time and break a quick sweat. If this is your thing, or could so, try it. After doing star jumps, or maybe going for a short run, a cigarette will probably be the last thing you'll want. You can also try 5 minutes of burpees or push-ups – anything that could render you a little out of breath and make your heart beat just a little faster. Or go and pull some weeds from your garden, reorganize your room, or clean the house. Do something to distract your mind and feel have you achieved something positive.

Drink water. If you have a craving, drink some water. This works for many people.

Overtime, you might find some of these thoughts and strategies work better than others. If they lose their effectiveness it is important to be creative and develop new strategies. It could be helpful to find a support group to share your story with and find inspiration from. Finding a support group is helpful regardless as you'll meet others who are going through the same experiences, have made it and actually stopped smoking. You could also go online and search for ideas and inspiration for distractions. Just be ready for your next craving and have something that works ready to go.

Chapter 6

Toxic People and Self-Doubt

You're slowly moving towards stopping smoking forever, but there's always going to be that voice that says "Once a smoker, always a smoker", or "Are you sure you're *never* going to have another cigarette?" That voice could be coming from you, or it could be coming from "toxic people." Toxic people, most often smokers (in this situation), will make you feel that stopping smoking is an impossible feat. They'll say or think things like "I stopped once for 4 years and started again – what makes you think you'll be able to do it?" Be wary of these people – more likely than not, they are saying these things because they don't want to be the only one left smoking, or be the one put to shame for continuing their habit. If they are close friends or relations, ask them to be supportive, and if they aren't, then stop being around them until you feel strong enough. The last thing you need is others infecting you with doubt.

Limit your social encounters with smokers unless you are confident that you can suppress the urge or craving to smoke when you see friends doing so, particularly if you're out at a bar and will be drinking alcohol. If you have close friends and partners who smoke, ask if they would like to stop together with you. If they aren't ready, you can help prepare them for it. Doing it together with friends or family could be immensely helpful; support each other throughout the experience and be strong together. If they aren't willing or wanting to quit, ask that they support you and try not to smoke when they're around you. If you're at a restaurant with others who smoke, ask them not to announce their cigarette breaks when they leave the table and not to leave together if there is more than one of them. Think of it this way: if they are true friends, who like or love you, then they should be supportive, just the same as you would be if they were stopping!

Dealing with external voices that cast doubt is easy enough; it's the self-doubt that you really have to try to overcome and cast aside. The key is to change the way you think about stopping. We have so much self-doubt. I believe that self-doubt stems from not experiencing something before – it's a fear of the unknown. For example, if you have never driven a car before you'll doubt that you can, but once you take your lessons and your confidence builds you start to realize that you can do it. Did you doubt that you could use a computer when you first sat down at one? It wasn't until you started to practice and use it that your self-doubt diminished and you were confident that you could do it. This way, slowly but surely, you start to believe in yourself, because you're actually doing it! It is the same with smoking; if you have never experienced being a Happy Non-Smoker, then you doubt you can be one. Once you do realize that you are becoming a Happy Non-Smoker, by cutting down at your pace, self-doubt will slowly dissipate.

Have you ever moved to a new address or worked in a new area and become lost, turned up on the wrong floor of a building, or gone to a shopping mall and forgotten where you'd left the car? We all have, but I bet with increased familiarity you became very adept at creating shortcuts and more comfortable in your surroundings. Stopping smoking is the same. Sometimes you need to "*get lost*" to get a better idea of where you are.

I realized that I doubted myself about things that I hadn't yet experienced in my life – like not smoking. It wasn't until I started to do it, by cutting down and realizing that I was stopping, that I started to believe in myself. I realized that I'd gone from twenty-five cigarettes per day to five per day in a matter of weeks; I didn't even really notice it happening. I thought *"I am doing it,"* and, in turn, this realization started to make me believe in myself. My doubt was diminishing and my power was rising. Don't think of it as quitting forever, because that, for most smokers, is a terrifying thought, and fear is not conducive to eliminating self-doubt. Instead, just think of it one moment at a time, one day at a time. "I'm not having this cigarette right now." Period. Don't think past it.

Not having that cigarette right now is something you *can* do. Remember, it's just three minutes. Remember all the thoughts and distractions you can use to overcome a craving. You don't have to let your inner doubt overpower you.

The French playwright and novelist Honoré de Balzac once wrote, *"When you doubt your power, you give power to your doubt."* Keep this in mind when you doubt your ability to stop smoking, or your ability to overcome cravings. The more you doubt yourself, the less confident you are and the harder stopping will be. Believe that you are strong enough to stop smoking, now, not later. Don't let your self-doubt strip away your logic and reason; keep believing in yourself, and believe that you can overcome this one craving.

Each time I attempted to stop smoking I always had a nagging feeling in the back of my mind that I could not do it. I hated it when Stop Smoking companies would tell you their success rates. "*We have a success rate of eighty percent.*" Well, as soon as I saw that, I automatically thought I would be in the twenty percent. This happened every time.

But there are times when no matter how hard you try to think positively, the self-doubt just lingers. You still feel sunken and defeated, like you can't stop yourself from having a cigarette, from succumbing to your craving. If this happens, you must confront your self-doubt. Ask yourself why you doubt yourself right now and what you're afraid of.

In my case, my greatest fear was that if I stopped smoking then I would never be able to have a cigarette ever again. This thought would make me shake and I'd become very upset. The way I got over this fear was to face it head on. I told myself that I was allowed to have a cigarette if I chose, just not right then at that moment, not when my body and mind were weak, which would help ease the pressure. Even though I never chose to smoke again, I knew that I could and that it wasn't forbidden. By giving myself that allowance and flexibility I was able to regain my composure and think of distractions once again in order to overcome that moment of craving or weakness.

When your inner voice, or a toxic person, is saying *"you're never going to be able to quit,"* just transform that doubt into a different question: *"What can I do right now to bring me closer to my want of stopping smoking?"* Take baby steps and think about 'right now', not some distant future. Be in the present.

If you need a confidence boost, don't think about the last time you had a cigarette or the last time you tried to stop and failed. Turn your attention to previous successes in your life. I know this can be hard; thinking of failures can be easier than thinking of successes and achievements we are proud of, but if you are having a self-doubt crisis then this is what you need. You need a boost in confidence; you need to know you have succeeded in the past with other endeavors, some of which are probably as challenging as not smoking, if not more. Write down your successes and keep the list with you; the next time you feel like you can't do this, pull it out and remind yourself how strong you really are. Some of these successes may be the beautiful children you've raised, the great rapport you have with people at work, or the great group of friends you have around you. Maybe it was when you were successful in obtaining your dream job. We all have successes in our lives and we need to recall and cherish them more than we do.

If there are toxic people around you, try to confront them (politely). And if they can't become supportive, then stop listening to them. You don't have to talk to them; you don't have to defend yourself. Toxic people try to suck away all of your good energy and willpower in order to put you down. Don't let them have the last laugh. If you stop listening to toxic people, it doesn't mean you have to cease being their friend or acquaintance, it just means that when it comes to smoking you're not going to hear what they have to say. Although, more generally speaking, toxic people are not good to have around in your life. They are inclined to take advantage of others' vulnerabilities and insecurities as a way of making themselves feel better and superior. Toxic people mirror your inner self-doubt; don't let their voice compound your inner voice, which you already have to address.

Toxic people might not always be blatantly toxic or unsupportive. They might not be casting doubt on you, smoking in front of you, or encouraging you to smoke again. They could be oblivious to their toxicity towards your efforts to stop.

Sometimes a toxic remark could be subtle and even unintentional. For example, you might say, *"I haven't had a cigarette in two weeks!"* Your inadvertent toxic commentator might say, *"Wait until you haven't had one in a month, you'll be even worse than you are now!"*

You need to catch that immediately. Don't let anyone force you into thinking about the future. Don't let them make you think about your greatest fear when it comes to being smoke-free. You have to address the problem right away:

"I thank you for how supportive you've been, but I'd really appreciate it if you could keep it to the now and not talk about the future. Talking about the future stresses me out and it makes me doubtful. Let's just talk about how

strong I am and how well I'm doing so far!"

Another example of the "undercover" toxic person is someone who might use scare tactics to help you. As I explained earlier, scare tactics do not work for many smokers. By now, if you've been reading this book, then you already know what you need to know about the harms of smoking. You don't need someone else using scare tactics and sending you videos of tarred lungs. When they do that, it could actually be subconsciously misconceived as doubt in your mind – you might feel like they don't believe that you can stop smoking or that you aren't strong enough to do it.

You might inadvertently think, *"Why are they sending me this? Because they think I need to be scared even more to stop?"* Don't let these subliminal messages affect your confidence. When you get these kinds of messages, face them head on. Talk to the person who sent you them and let them know that you're aware of the harms of smoking, and that you're stopping smoking because you want to be healthier. Tell them that scare tactics only make you doubt yourself more, which is the last thing you need right now.

Toxic people and negative comments will come up

during your quest. Be prepared and know how to address them:

- Tell a toxic person right away that they're being unsupportive and aren't helping you with your quest. (Don't use these words exactly, but think of a polite way to say it without putting them down. Don't call them toxic.). My health and wellbeing are more important than some relationships I might have.

- Don't defend yourself – you don't need to. Defending yourself could lead to increased self-doubt and insecurity.

- Explain to them what they did or said could be toxic.

- Give them alternatives, things they can do or say that would be supportive to help you stay strong.

- If a person you've previously addressed is persistently toxic, then you should disengage and stop being around them, at least while you're stopping smoking.

Be proactive about your social environment; you have power and control over how you deal with your want to stop smoking. If comments or actions of another triggers self-doubt or a craving episode, try and identify the exact cause and address it. Don't let it go by and hope it won't happen again – in other words, don't be reactive; be proactive in your efforts. Immediately address the situation to make sure it doesn't happen again.

If you feel some people around you aren't providing support, or that you just need extra support to get through the toughest moments during this journey, look for support groups or maybe even a personal coach. That's what I did. It might only take one toxic comment to set you off – just be aware. I started a support group in my home town and invited people along who wanted to stop smoking. Being able to talk to me as well as others in the group helped these people immensely.

If trying to stop smoking entirely on your own seems almost impossible; then external support is extremely important. When I first began the process to stop I found I had nobody to talk to and really needed some extra help. I ended up seeking the service of a personal coach, Michael Nitti, who became a key contributor to my success. Michael taught me that it was my mind that craved the nicotine. By this point, I had already spent about a month working on stopping smoking, but was still smoking quite a few cigarettes per day. He told me that my mind didn't want to let me stop smoking because it was in survival mode. I'd been smoking for so long that my mind thought it was something I needed in order to survive when, in reality, my body knew otherwise.

Michael encouraged me to believe in myself, to believe I could really stop. One of his methods for overcoming self-doubt is setting small goals every day, goals that are attainable. Each time I achieved a goal I would feel stronger and more confident. These didn't necessarily have to be goals related to smoking; they were just meant to help maintain or boost my confidence and to ensure I didn't become overwhelmed by self-doubt. For example, a goal might be to cook a healthy meal each night – I'd achieve it and feel *good*. Another goal was to start running up hills. When I went for my runs I would visualize myself running up them before I got there. Once I had completed the run I had fulfilled my visualization, thereby reinforcing my self-belief. I would start to believe that I could do the task at hand and eventually, I actually did it. Michael told me to concentrate on the accomplishments, however big or small, to make my goals happen, and to praise myself for achieving them. This is the "Trophy Effect," which Michael wrote a book about (www.trophyeffect.com).

As adults, we are very bad at giving ourselves praise. We only seem to criticize ourselves for our faults and slip-ups. We need to start praising ourselves more and criticizing less. Look at young children – they applaud themselves for each and every small achievement.

Chapter 7

Reward Yourself for Stopping

Every cigarette you don't smoke is an achievement – it's that simple.

A good way to move yourself closer towards your 'want' to stop smoking, is to reward yourself along the way. In fact, it's almost impossible to stay on track to stopping if you don't regularly reward yourself. Rewarding yourself recognizes your efforts as well as your strengths; it reinforces your confidence and self-belief.

Addiction is based on a reward system – you become addicted to things and develop habits that give you pleasure and reward, and you become fearful of things you associate with bad outcomes. It's the basis of psychological conditioning – think Pavlov's dog.

The bulk of the last few chapters has been about the bad stuff: dealing with toxic people and self-doubt, trying to associate real harms of smoking with the habit of smoking, and trying to disassociate yourself from environments and habits that are related to smoking. This chapter is about developing a reward system for breaking the addiction and breaking the habit. If you associate stopping with something good – something immediately good – then your chances of succeeding will increase infinitely.

Smoking itself is often associated with rewards. Yes, nicotine actually activates our brain's "reward pathways" by mimicking dopamine and stimulating your dopamine receptors. When dopamine is released, it makes you feel good. Other activities that stimulate dopamine release (the real dopamine, not a fake, mimicked form of dopamine) include having sex and exercising. Without sufficient dopamine, you can become sluggish and depressed, which is part of the reason why nicotine withdrawal can sometimes lead to depression. As a regular smoker, your body has become used to getting a nicotine kick throughout the day, which makes you feel good, just like dopamine. When you stop smoking, suddenly there's no more nicotine and your body reacts to it – it's tricked into thinking there isn't enough dopamine because it got used to all the nicotine. As a result, you may start becoming depressed or unmotivated.

This could hurt your efforts to stop!

You don't want to feel uninterested in life; you need to feel good about yourself in order to succeed (in anything), and that includes stopping smoking. Foods like almonds, avocados, bananas, low-fat dairy, meat and poultry, lima beans, and sesame and pumpkin seeds may all help your body to produce more dopamine.

It is important to replace the nicotine with alternatives to trigger a release of dopamine. Yes, you could have more sex, perhaps – but that might not always be practical. You can't have sex every time you have a craving! Instead, you have to come up with a reward system, one that gradually goes from very frequent but small rewards to less frequent but larger rewards. Your body will reach a natural equilibrium and will no longer think it needs the nicotine. Eventually you'll be back with dopamine only, which is more than enough and is our natural state.

The rewards of smoking are more than purely physiological. They also come in social and psychological forms. For example, you might smoke while socializing (more so when alcohol is involved) and having fun with your friends – that's a rewarding experience in itself.

You need to recognize that none of this is real. The physiological part is just forgery – the nicotine is only pretending to be dopamine, something that makes you think you feel good when in fact it's harming you silently, slowly. The social part is just a masquerade – hanging out with friends and socializing are fun activities; you don't need smoking to make them better! Nicotine doesn't come with any *real* rewards, but rather with an endless list of harms and life-long penalties.

So let's rejig and shake up your system. We started this journey by discussing about how to break routines and habits, how to disrupt the existing reward associations. Now it's time to set up a new reward system associated with stopping, an easy reward system could be a financial one. Smoking is an expensive and inconvenient habit – in the developed world, each pack can cost up to $15, and that amount is only going to increase. If you smoke a pack a day, that's $105 a week and $420 a month. What can you treat yourself to with $15 a day? You could go to a movie – there's no smoking there. You could treat yourself to a nice meal. And for $420 you can treat yourself to a full-day spa retreat, a couple of nights in a luxury motel, or even a better car or house to live in. Save that money for a couple more months, and you've got yourself a flight and hotel package to a resort somewhere to escape winter. If you're a casual worker, you could cut back your hours at work to spend more time with your children.

Setting up a financial reward system can show you immediately what you are saving by not smoking. It can also help you become healthier in other ways – every time you treat yourself you're also improving your general wellbeing. If the reward is a drop-in yoga class or a spa day, it's pretty obvious how that will make you healthier. But even if it's not something so obvious, any little treat that makes you happier will lead to better health outcomes – that's just the way our bodies work. Happy thoughts lead to a healthier you, while negative thoughts make you less healthy and more susceptible to disease.

When it comes to setting up your financial reward system, you don't actually have to physically save up the money somewhere. You can always tally it on your computer or in a logbook of some sort – just keep track of it! While you are keeping track of the money saved, start brainstorming different things that you want or would like to do and mark down how much they would cost. These could be activities or goods, they could be items you already have but want more of, they could be things you already do but want to do more of, or they could be anything that makes you feel good. After you have accomplished this list, you can decide what you want to treat yourself to first. Start with something small so that you don't have to wait too long before you get a reward – pick something worth the value of a pack of cigarettes. Do that at least a few times before you start moving towards larger rewards. The larger the reward, the longer you'll have to wait, so make sure you're ready for that!

Besides the benefit of treating yourself, the financial reward system could also give you motivation when you have doubts or cravings. For example:

"If I can just make it to tomorrow without buying a pack, then I can go get a ten minute massage!"

"If I can just make it for a week, I'll have enough money to buy those really cool running shoes I've always wanted!"

As with everything else we've discussed, each person needs to create his or her own reward system based on their interests and personality. For me, sometimes a movie or a simple pat on the back was enough. Finding little, neat activities that you truly appreciate but rarely get to enjoy, is an easy way to reward yourself during this journey.

Here are some tips for setting up a good rewards system:

- Don't just go with the flow and come up with rewards as you go along. Set up the system in advance so you have things to look forward to and activities to motivate you when you feel discouraged. Write down what you'd really like.

- Set up reward levels and benchmarks. Start by rewarding yourself every time you overcome a craving. Decide how long you want to reward yourself at this benchmark and with what, before moving on to the next level, which could be for every day, and again decide the rewards and the time span, and so on. Be "giving" when you set up these levels and benchmarks; set up more rewards than necessary for longer periods of time than you think you'll need at each level. Make sure you have significantly more small rewards than larger rewards. If you feel that you no longer require rewards at a certain level and there are more rewards still, just move on to the next level anyway and get the better rewards!

- Make sure your rewards are meaningful to you. For some, goods or monetary rewards – a new pair of shoes, for example – are suitable, but for others, reward activities might work better. For example, treating yourself to some alone time with some music and a good book could be more rewarding than buying something for yourself. Buying gifts for your children or grandchildren might give you pleasure also.

- Your rewards might not have to do only with how long you've stopped; they could also be for specific challenges you've overcome or other habits you've broken. For example, for every time you don't smoke while out with friends who are smokers, give yourself a reward! Reward yourself for the toughest habits and routines, the toughest associations.

- As was mentioned earlier, it isn't wise to replace smoking with food. That also means not rewarding yourself with food. You don't want to open another can of worms. Chewing sugar-free gum is a good option.

- While on this topic: don't reward yourself with a cigarette! This might seem trivial and obvious, but trust me, it will come up. You might have just met a huge deadline and think, "What's better than a cigarette to celebrate?" Or worse still, you might reward yourself with a cigarette because you haven't had any cigarettes for a period of time. "I haven't had one in so long!" We always want the forbidden fruit. But just think – there are *other* forbidden fruits that you also want; think about what those might be and reward yourself with one of them.

- Don't forget why you are being rewarded. Be sure that each reward marks an achievement in your progress towards being smoke-free.

- Prepare to celebrate your eventual success. Stopping smoking altogether is a tremendous victory, and needs to be celebrated. Plan what your celebration will be – a trip to Europe, perhaps? Once you've made this plan, solidify it by sharing it with others. Tell them so they can be excited for you as well!

Once you've created this new reward system, stopping will become that much easier.

Chapter 8

The Biggest Challenges When Stopping

Anyone who has ever tried to stop smoking will be familiar with some of the challenges. This chapter will discuss some of the biggest challenges I faced during my journey and how I overcame them. Hopefully this will also help prepare you for some of the challenges you might face in your own efforts to stop. Some of what I'm about to talk about will seem familiar to you because I might have discussed it before, but familiarity with the upcoming challenges and possible solutions is important to being successful.

Relapsing

I must admit, when I began to stop smoking (for the thirteenth and final time) I didn't really believe that I could do it, as I was never strong enough before during every other attempt. As I discussed in Chapter 6, I did end up believing in myself, after my coach guided me towards overcoming any self-doubt I experienced along the way. I overpowered and destroyed my self-doubt. I realized I had to be strong.

With strength comes perseverance. If you don't persevere in your efforts to get something that you don't have, but want, then you won't end up getting it. That is true of everything in life, as we all know.

Because I did relapse on several occasions when I was stopping smoking, I had to practice and learn how to get back on track again. Instead of doubting myself, I would think of ways to do it better the next time. Was my reward system not meaningful enough? Was I not finding good enough distractions to suppress my cravings? How could I make it work for the next attempt? Like anyone else who has ever fallen, I had to get up, brush myself off, and start again. I reminded myself each time I relapsed that this was just a practice run. The more I practiced stopping, the better I'd get at it. And eventually, it would happen. And it did. As children, when we fell off our bicycles there was never a second thought about getting back on and continuing to practice until we succeeded.

I always knew that trying to stop smoking was going to be challenging. But I also knew that life would be even harder than this if I didn't stop now. In the long run, if I didn't stop, who knew what sort of health problems I might develop, and how difficult and painful just living day to day might become. So I kept persevering and I finally achieved the outcome I was going after: to not be dependent on nicotine, to be a "happy" non-smoker. We have to keep persevering to stop; that is the key. This might take months, it might even take years, but wouldn't you rather have started now and not waited for another five to ten years? The sooner you start trying to stop, the more health gains you can make in the long run. Remind yourself of the timeline of good things that happen to your body over time as you cut cigarettes out of your life, and also remember that the longer you smoke, the more irreversible damage the smoking will do to your body. Each additional cigarette counts, and each additional cigarette you *don't* smoke also counts.

Jealousy

One thing I found at the beginning was how jealous I would be of other people who were still smoking. I would even use this as an excuse for myself: "If they're smoking, why can't I?" But when I thought more deeply about my jealousy, I knew that it actually wasn't real. I knew they weren't actually enjoying those cigarettes – it was all in my mind. And if I watched more closely, I knew that I was right. I saw them trying to hide behind buildings to get out of the way of kids and adults who gave them stares. I saw them duck out of restaurants in negative temperatures, shivering while puffing away at their cigarettes by themselves. I saw them trapped inside smoking rooms in airports with all the other smokers, hurriedly finishing up their "needed" smokes so they could get out of there. I had been in those situations many times, and I knew I didn't want to have to be in them ever again.

You definitely go through a metamorphosis when you stop smoking. It's like accomplishing the impossible. I had *never* experienced this before. You really do feel stronger and you feel like you can do anything. I know there are no limits to what I can accomplish as long as I set my mind to it, I prepare for it, and I'm ready to persevere. After nearly two years of not smoking this feeling is normal for me now. The craving for a cigarette does rear its ugly head sometimes, but now I know how to handle that situation: by acknowledging the feeling and not trying to fight it.

Identity Crisis

I also felt like I was going through an identity crisis. Being a non-smoker was very foreign to me and it took quite a while to get use to my new identity. I felt like an imposter at the beginning.

Feeling Alienated

I felt like I was the only person in the world trying to become nicotine-free, even though this wasn't true. But I felt alone. That is when I sought the help of a personal coach, after trying all other avenues. I really am proud of myself for being strong, especially when I was seeking out inspiration and encouragement. In the beginning I really did need *someone* to talk to. I tried to find smoking groups, but to no avail. I even phoned Narcotics Anonymous (NA) to see if I could go to their meetings. They said I could, but I chickened out because I thought I might not fit in.

I overcame this challenge by seeking professional help, but there are also many other options you could try out as well. We've already discussed many of them, including seeking out support groups and including your other friends and colleagues who smoke in your journey. Stopping smoking together with close friends could help you feel supported and encouraged, and you wouldn't have to feel like you were fighting this battle alone. As I suggested in an earlier chapter, why not start up a challenge at work and have a prize for the person who is smoking the fewest cigarettes after a certain period of time?

Trigger Areas

Trigger areas are everywhere: the patio of a bar you always visit, the room or area in your house where you always smoke, or the bus stop where you always have a cigarette while you wait. For me, within my own home, there was only one spot where I used to smoke. This was a big trigger area for me, so when I started cutting down on my smoking, I never smoked in that area and I made it a smoke-free zone. We also moved the furniture around in our indoor living area just to make a small difference to my usual surroundings. I disrupted the association, and now I can be in that area without thinking of smoking. It is a relief to sit there without constantly being reminded of smoking. When you are trying to find different places to smoke instead of your trigger areas, try to find places that you don't frequent. When you are smoking at home, smoke around the back of your house or somewhere that you don't go often and can't see from the area of the house where you entertain. If you're going to smoke at a bus stop, go to one that is far away and that you won't go to again. You don't want to create new trigger areas in places you often frequent.

Becoming Irritated and Other Symptoms of Nicotine Withdrawal

I must admit that I did become irritable at times while stopping. When this happened, I just had to remind myself of the reasons why I wasn't smoking. The importance and benefits of stopping far outweighed the unpleasantness of being mad for a minute. I also warned people in my family and others who were close to me that I would probably go through some irritability. This way, they were able to be prepared and when it happened they could help soothe my frustrations by being supportive and providing encouraging and motivating words. Irritation, frustration, and anger associated with nicotine withdrawal usually don't last very long though. By two to four weeks after stopping these feelings do disappear.

Other symptoms you might encounter include: anxiety or nervousness, difficulty concentrating, restlessness and insomnia, headaches, fatigue, increased coughing, constipation or upset stomach, tremors, and depression. This seems like a big list, but remember: none of these symptoms last very long. They are all temporary. Remember, you smoked for decades, so some discomfort for a couple of weeks isn't a great inconvenience. Tremors, constipation, and upset stomach usually only last one to two weeks. Insomnia, fatigue, restlessness, and headaches usually last between two and four weeks. Difficulty concentrating, depression, and coughing could last for a few to several weeks. I only point this out so that you know that you're normal if and when these symptoms occur. We seem to be scared that these things will happen to us when we stop getting nicotine, but we don't seem to care about the negative health effects of actually smoking cigarettes. (Quite ironic little creatures, aren't we?)

If at any point you feel like these symptoms are overwhelming you and you are feeling extremely helpless, don't give in – get extra help.

Trying to Find Replacements for Smoking

I had a really tough time finding suitable replacements

for smoking. This was especially true when it came to the cravings associated with my emotions. When I was stressed about work, or was really tired, the first thing I wanted was a cigarette. When I felt like taking a short break from strenuous work, I wanted a cigarette. These emotions were often the cause of the relapses during my previous attempts to stop.

I knew I needed to find ways to address those feelings, since they weren't things I could avoid, so I sat down and took some time to really identify why I thought a cigarette could help. Then I dispelled that association. By thinking this through I was able to reinforce in my mind that a cigarette wouldn't actually help in dealing with or resolving any of the stress and anxiety. If anything, it would make me worse, because as soon as I finished one cigarette I wanted to have another one. There are much more effective ways to deal with these feelings, but I had to learn about them. I had spent too much time in my life using cigarettes as my life-support; I needed healthy ways to address my emotions. I really focused on what I was gaining by stopping, and I started to practice breathing exercises – taking a long, deep breath and counting to three, and then letting it out slowly, again counting to three. These newly learned activities helped to center me; they helped me to re-focus on my wants. They calmed my nerves and helped relax me, much more effectively than any cigarette could have ever done.

If you can't find ways to help deal with emotional triggers for smoking, then you might have to learn about new ones, like I did. There are many strategies out there that could be perfect replacements for cigarettes when you face those triggers.

There are going to be many challenges you face along the way, and you might lose to some of them and relapse. When this happens, not only is it important to pick yourself right back up and start again, but it is also crucial to be mindful of why the relapse happened. Pay attention to what the challenge was and write down important triggers related to it. Was it the people you were with or what you were doing? Was it because of where you were or what you were feeling?

Once you've written these things down, start brainstorming strategies for how to handle the challenge the next time it arises. Try learning new techniques and activities that might be directly related to that challenge. Challenges are never completely unique – it is always possible to find someone else who experienced a similar challenge and beat it, and it is always possible to find solutions and strategies you weren't aware of before. You just have to look for them; don't lose faith too easily.

Chapter 9

Challenge the Smoking Justifications

It's been weeks, or months, or even years since you stopped smoking and you feel great about yourself. But still, the thought of a cigarette will pop into your mind. That feeling of inhaling a deep breath of smoke, and the lingering taste, might be just what you want. By now, stopping has become second nature to you. You can now accept and acknowledge that craving, and you know it's just a thought that will pass, like any other thought. And it does.

Sometimes, though, that thought might persist. You could be going through a really stressful time in your life – that can be a huge trigger leading many people to turn back to smoking.

Because we are brainwashed into thinking that smoking has so many benefits, we come up with justifications to continue smoking, or to start again after we have stopped. Here are some of the common justifications:

"I enjoy smoking so much."

You don't enjoy inhaling cigarette smoke – you enjoy the effects of nicotine and the deep breaths you take when you are smoking. That is why you smoke. If you enjoy smoking so much, would you encourage your children or grandchildren to join you in having a cigarette? I don't think so. If you enjoyed surfing or playing cards, then you would encourage them to join you.

"We all have to die from something."

I know I would rather die peacefully in my sleep than in pain in a hospital with no dignity.

"I might get hit by a bus tomorrow."

If you get lung cancer, you will probably feel like you did get hit by a bus. The chances of you getting hit by a bus are very slim, but the chances of you getting a smoking-related disease are very real – remember, one in two, or fifty percent. I'd like those odds on any horse race but not on my life.

"I'm very stressed at the moment."

This is probably the *most* used excuse for smoking in all of history. People who don't smoke get stressed too, but they don't reach for a cigarette. They take deep breaths and sit down and think about the problem logically, or take a break from whatever they are doing and go for a walk, do some stretching or meditating, listen to music, or find a friend or loved one to be with. They are able to find ways to deal with the stress, which could include seeking professional help. These methods are also available to smokers, but they choose to smoke instead.

Remember, smoking actually creates stress. We've already described how nicotine mimics dopamine, and what happens when your body thinks it's running out of dopamine – it gets stressed, among other things. So the more you smoke, the more often you're going to suffer from nicotine withdrawal symptoms, which can appear within an hour of not smoking. This leads to more stress over time, and more anxiety.

Imagine a smoker and a non-smoker in a meeting for a long time, or taking a long-haul flight from Australia to New York. Who do you think will have the most anxiety and stress about their situation? The smoker will be a lot more stressed than the non-smoker. I am sure that once you succeed in handling a single stressful situation without grabbing a cigarette, and instead resolve it via different means, you will have the confidence necessary to succeed many times over.

Just remember that there are other, more effective ways than smoking to deal with stress and stress-causing situations, and if you have managed to do it once before then remind yourself of this fact and know that you can do so again. More often than not, smoking a cigarette is just an excuse to take a break, or maybe go outside. So do that – go outside, take a walk, take a few deep breaths of fresh air, and enjoy the outside without having to poison yourself with more toxic chemicals.

"I smoke when I am bored."

Often smokers will turn to cigarettes or, rather, to nicotine when they're bored. It might be that a smoker is waiting to meet someone or for a bus, or maybe he or she is working on something tedious. But cigarettes don't actually make you any less bored – they really, actually don't. You don't smoke because you are bored – you smoke to break up the monotony! So if you get bored while waiting, have something with you at all times that you enjoy, like a good book, a collection of sudoku's or crossword puzzles, or some fun games on your phone. All of these small, little activities will be much more effective at resolving your boredom than smoking, which does nothing except reduce your health. Additionally, these other activities also happen to make you feel good, without making you sick.

Try to come up with handy things that you can do to break the monotony anywhere and at any time, so that boredom can no longer be an excuse for smoking.

Try this experiment: mimic having a cigarette, the same way you would have one if you were bored. Mimic having one with a pen or straw, and see how many inhalations you actually complete. I bet you only do about three inhalations because it is *so boring*!

"I like to have a cigarette when I drink."

Many people associate smoking with drinking. If you're a smoker, you're more likely to smoke more heavily when drinking alcohol. The most basic reason for this is that the consumption of alcohol leads to a gradual loss of self-control.

People who are irritable tend to become more aggressive when they drink alcohol. People who are sad or depressed will be even more visibly affected by their sadness when they are intoxicated. So if you're a smoker trying to cut down or stop, you will probably have much less control over your smoking whilst drinking alcohol. In this situation, it is *really* difficult to come up with logical reasons for why you shouldn't satisfy your craving or your urge to have another puff.

Don't let that be you. All smokers *think* that cutting out cigarettes smoked when drinking is perhaps one of the toughest things to do, but you can make it happen. The first step is to cut out the drinking – you don't necessarily need to do this completely, but maybe just don't allow yourself to become inebriated. If you find that you really can't fight the urge to smoke whenever you have a drink, no matter how hard you try to distract yourself, don't drink at all. If you relapse because of drinking, take note of how much you drank – and cut back. Don't drink more until you are sure you are ready to take on that challenge.

Mind you, though, drinking might not be a smoking trigger for everyone. For me, it wasn't at all. When I was stopping, I found it the easiest to not have a cigarette when I was drinking – enjoying my friends' company and talking with them actually worked as my distraction.

"I'm putting on weight."

Nicotine withdrawal can sometimes feel like hunger pangs. If you put on weight, it's very likely because you have chosen to replace cigarettes with food or have decided to reward yourself with food. If you do gain weight, that's not a reason to start smoking again. Putting on a few pounds, or maybe even more, is less concerning than smoking more. You can lose those pounds by being healthier, but you might not be able to reverse some of the negative effects of smoking.

Try to keep track of your diet and identify how it has changed since you stopped smoking. Once you've done that, you can then properly develop a strategy for avoiding overeating. Furthermore, now that you have put away the cigarettes you can try out new exercises and activities that might have been limited by your smoking before.

"I have to smoke after a meal."

The post-meal cigarette is really common for smokers. One of the reasons why (beyond it being a ritual habit) is that nicotine stimulates your digestive system – and not in

a good way. This is also why one of the symptoms of nicotine withdrawal is indigestion; it's because your digestive
system slows down when you stop smoking.

But don't let that fool you. The smoking is doing abso-
lutely no good for your digestion. Smoking actually con-
tributes to common disorders such as heartburn and pep-
tic ulcers. It also increases the risk of some diseases in your
digestive system, including Crohn's disease (an inflamma-
tory bowel disease). Your digestion will be better in the
long run if you stop smoking.

Here is a nice way to overcome after-meal cravings
that worked for me: try inviting some friends who don't
smoke over for dinner. Pay attention to how they act after
a meal and ask yourself, "Why don't they need to smoke?"
If you are craving a cigarette after a meal, take some deep
breaths to help relax your body and consider going for a
walk to help metabolize the food. Remember, we weren't
born smokers, so our natural digestive system works just
fine without nicotine.

"Smoking helps me concentrate."

Nicotine is a stimulant and, in the short-term, it does

increase alertness and therefore can help you concentrate. But in the long-term nicotine also acts as a depressant and once the initial rush goes away you become more lethargic than you were before the cigarette. This is why nicotine withdrawal symptoms include difficulty concentrating.

But again, you have to find other ways to concentrate. This could mean taking a quick break (without smoking), talking to someone about your work or something else, or thinking of a reward to motivate you and help you concentrate.

Within a few weeks of stopping smoking, your ability to focus and concentrate will return to normal. Don't let the withdrawal symptoms lure you back into smoking. We're just hitting the reboot button when we allow nicotine to leave our bodies and go back to our natural state.

"I'm not sick, so I don't need to stop."

I wasn't sick (apart from my terrible cough), but that's why I stopped. I thought that I had pushed the envelope as much as I could and that it was time to take responsibility for my own well-being. We all need to be responsible for ourselves and ensure that we can live a healthy, pain-free life and not end up in a hospital bed struggling to breathe. Try this experiment: take your pulse before and after you smoke. Notice how fast your heart beats after you smoke. Imagine this happening each time you have a cigarette, wearing out your heart and putting unnecessary stress on your cardiovascular system. The idea is to stop before you *do* get sick, because you eventually will as a result of smoking.

"There is too much going on in my life at the moment."

"Don't wait; the time will never be just right." – Napoleon Hill, American author of *'Think and Grow Rich'*.

Ready! Fire! Aim! – that's right, fire before you aim; you can always sort the aiming out after you've fired, but if you never fire you won't ever succeed. There's never going to be a perfect day to stop smoking. Don't put it off because you think there will be a perfect day. Start by cutting down; you don't have to think of this as quitting. Just take it one step at a time. This is better than not starting to stop at all. The end result will be worth it. Remember: if you change nothing, nothing will change.

"I don't want to become a "reformed" smoker."

As smokers we all hate the "reformed smoker". The guy who is constantly screwing his nose up at you and waving his hands at the cigarette smoke. Telling you, *"you shouldn't smoke you know"*. We have no time for these people and fear that we will become one if we stop smoking, because some of the ex-smokers we know have become reformed smokers. I am not a reformed smoker. I only try to help other people who want to stop. You could also do this when you finally become free. Having someone to talk to while you go through the process is invaluable and you could be that person for someone else. What a great way to reinforce your decision to stop!

"I feel like a cigarette."

You may feel like a cigarette, but you don't need one. Just accept the feeling and move on. You don't have to have one, just because you feel like one.

You now have everything you need to start to stop smoking. Let's run through the checklist:

✓ You have *'your'* plan for becoming nicotine free.

✓ You've created a list of thoughts and ideas that can help turn you off smoking when you most feel you need to.

✓ You can change your environment to reduce temptation.

✓ You can reward yourself for your efforts and progress, as well as congratulating yourself for every small achievement.

✓ You are able to reject any negativity from external sources, as well as any of your own negative thoughts.

✓ You've come up with a myth-buster for every justification in the book.

✓ You persevere and deal with any setbacks.

You just have to *believe* that you can. And you also have to start referring to yourself as a non-smoker. "Would you like a smoke?" "No, I'm a non-smoker."

Chapter 10

The Joys of Being a Non-Smoker

Anyone who's ever stopped smoking will tell you that it's the greatest thing they've done. And I won't tell you otherwise. Not only is it a huge achievement, but it's also the best thing to do for your body.

It's been nearly two years since I had my last cigarette. That might not seem long to some toxic people, but I know for sure that I won't be going back. I could have waited 5 years to write and publish this book, but I want to start helping people now, and I know all the things I can do, all the right strategies to use, if I ever feel like I have an excuse to take a puff. That just won't happen.

When you are still a smoker, fear is your worst enemy – the fear of failing, the fear of not ever having a smoke again, the fear of all the challenges you'll face when hanging out with other smokers. But once you've overcome that, moved to the other side of the fence, and become a non-smoker, that fear doesn't exist anymore. Instead, what you feel is relief and joy.

- ✓ You are no longer encumbered by having to stock up on smokes before that road trip.
- ✓ You no longer have to stand outside in the frigid cold

to have that cigarette.

✓ You no longer have to trap yourself in confined designated smoking rooms just to get that hit of nicotine.

✓ You no longer get out of breath just from walking up a flight of stairs.

✓ You no longer have phlegm coughs every morning.

✓ You no longer reek of stale smoke when you're in a room or a small space.

✓ You no longer have to buy cigarettes.

✓ You no longer have to panic if you have run out of cigarettes.

If you want it bad enough, this could be you too. Learn to reroute any self-doubt, don't listen to toxic people, and learn to address excuses and triggers. We've talked about almost everything. And if ever you feel lost, know that you aren't alone.

Just imagine what it would mean to you and your family and how proud you would be if you could tell people that you are a non-smoker.

I've stopped smoking for nearly two years now. According to the statistics, this means that:

- ✓ My blood pressure and pulse are normal;

- ✓ My circulation is perfectly normal, as is the temperature of my hands and feet;

- ✓ The carbon monoxide and oxygen levels in my blood are consistently normal;

- ✓ I no longer have any nicotine withdrawal symptoms;

- ✓ I have an excellent sense of taste and smell that far exceeds what it was when I was smoking;

- ✓ I have zero cravings;

- ✓ I no longer have a chronic cough, morning, night, or at all;

- ✓ My risk of heart disease is now half that of a current smoker; and

- ✓ Soon enough, without even being conscious of it, my risk of heart disease, stroke, and death from lung cancer will be the same as that of people who have never smoked.

I even love life more than before. Once you have successfully become nicotine free, you realize that you can do anything.

Knowing all of this makes me proud, and it continues to motivate me. I feel much healthier and have become much more active since my last cigarettes. I've stopped worrying about every little ache or pain or twinge in my body because I've stopped smoking.

I hope that my journey and experience, as well as this book, will help you move towards your own goals of stopping smoking.

Even now, if you are not ready to stop smoking all together, start cutting back on the cigarettes you smoke each day. This doesn't take much effort on your part and your mind and body will gradually get used to smoking less. Believe me, I know this happens.

I served twenty-seven years in nicotine jail and paid up to six thousand dollars per year, or seventy thousand dollars overall, for the privilege of being an inmate.

It is such a relief to have that proverbial monkey off my back. I was always quite healthy, exercised regularly, and ate well, but I always had smoking in the back of my mind. I was doing everything else right, except for that. Now I go for a jog and I no longer have to feel embarrassed by my breathing.

I removed the illusions of smoking. Smoking wasn't enjoyable. I only wanted the nicotine, not the cigarette. The day I realized I never wanted to smoke again was the best day of my *life*!!!! When you're addicted you have no idea how much you have to bow down to cigarettes. You are so free when that noose has finally been taken from around your throat.

I've found I do more things now, and take up more opportunities than when I smoked, because I no longer fear going somewhere where I won't be able to smoke.

I am always focusing on what I've gained, not the loss of smoking. The only thing I lost due to stopping smoking was a terrible cough. I have gained money, health, freedom, and respect. I find now that a lot of people do respect me for not smoking anymore. Non-smokers don't understand why people smoke; they are perplexed by this and respect you more when you don't. I know one thing: I'm not putting any more money into the coffers of the tobacco companies. I now have that money for myself.

I have finally accomplished what all smokers want to accomplish – to *never smoke again* – and it feels *fantastic*! I am so grateful that I don't need to smoke ever again.

We all know that we need to stop smoking sooner or later. If we don't stop for ourselves, smoking will stop us once and for all. Wouldn't you rather choose your destiny, instead of letting nicotine choose it for you?

Like a smoker once said to me when he had started to stop: "Us smokers, we're a dying breed." I couldn't agree more.

Conclusion

I never thought in a million years that I would stop smoking. Just like you think it won't happen for you. Give it a go; give your mind and your body time to get used to the idea. It is going to happen eventually so you may as well start now. What are you waiting for? Are you waiting until you do get a disease and maybe then you will HAVE to stop? Do you really think that a disease will have any effect on you? Unless of course you are bed bound in hospital and you can't smoke. Wouldn't you like to start now and know that you are one day closer to stopping forever?

Like I said in my Youtube video, I want to help as many people to become non-smokers, so we can then ALL help other smokers stop. I want you to help me, as I can't do it all on my own. I need extra help from people like you who will also become happy non-smokers, the sooner the better. Don't put up with nicotine controlling your life anymore. Take action today and take back control of your life.

To not smoke cigarettes anymore will be the best thing that you have ever done. Ask any ex-smoker and they will tell you exactly the same. As I said earlier, you will be healthier and wealthier, but the biggest reward is FREEDOM. No more slavery to the poison that has controlled your life for decades.

Remember you are not making a sacrifice when you stop smoking. You are making a sacrifice if you continue to smoke. This is the ultimate sacrifice – your life!

DOWNLOAD YOUR BONUS!

Simply go to:

www.saveyourbreathbook.com

www.ingramcontent.com/pod-product-compliance
Lightning Source LLC
Chambersburg PA
CBHW072156270326
41930CB00011B/2446